SLEEP TO WIN

SKYROCKETING YOUR PRODUCTIVITY BY SLEEPING BETTER

DELANEY WILDE

INTRODUCTION

TABLE OF CONTENT

SLEEP TO WIN

SKYROCKETING YOUR PRODUCTIVITY BY SLEEPING BETTER

INTRODUCTION

According to Aristotle, one of the founding fathers of ancient philosophy, we are the products of our daily habits. Excellence, then, was not an act, but a habit. The average entrepreneur, professional, college student or worker in the 21st century has an extremely demanding lifestyle. Now, more than ever before, we have so much to do, and it never seems like we can ever get enough time to carry out all our responsibilities. Maintaining a work-life balance has never been so difficult. Why exactly is the life of the average 21st-century individual so seemingly grueling?

Logically, our lives are actually supposed to be easier than the lives of the people who lived in previous generations. Technology has never been this advanced. We have mobile phones for instant communication, washing machines for the laundry, microwave cookers to warm our foods, refrigerators to store our food, virtual assistants to remind us of tasks ahead…technology has assisted us, in more ways than we can imagine to make our lives easier, but somehow, this current generation of students, workers and professionals seem to be the most stressed out, ever. How have we gotten it wrong?

The answer is that we are allowing the same technology that is supposed to save us, to enslave us. Instead of getting enough sleep, resting to rejuvenate our bodies and minds to gear up for the next day's activities, we stay up late at night, roaming all over social media, watching TV series on Netflix, or watching music videos on YouTube. No generation before us has ever had the chance to be extremely and consistently productive as we can actually be, but no generation before us has also had to deal with so many distractions. Now, it boils down to exactly how we want to use the gift of technology – to liberate ourselves, or to keep ourselves in perpetual stagnation or even regression?

A lot of people in today's competitive world desire to have an impact on people; to have their voices heard. Hence, both online and offline, a lot of people are becoming inspirational and motivational speakers. Now, I personally do not have a problem with motivational speakers. As a matter of fact, I spend a good chunk of my time per week listening to amazing podcasts on self-development and inculcation of productivity-enhancing habits. A lot of the inspirational and motivational material I consume online and offline actually do encourage me to take calculated risks, take leaps of faith, and leave fear behind. However, the problem with the internet is that it makes it possible for different people from different backgrounds and with different ideologies to pass information across to a potentially unlimited audience. And that's a very dangerous opportunity that has proven to be disastrous in a lot of cases.

All over YouTube, Instagram, Twitter, and Facebook, you'll find several videos telling you to go for your goals, to crush life, to sleep by 1 am and wake up at 4 am! WHAT? What normal human being expects to survive and perform optimally on just 3 hours or less of sleep? The sad thing is that people are consuming these misguiding content extremely ravenously, and it's not only having devastating effects on their health, it's also terribly affecting their productivity, performance and career growth. The truth is that getting less sleep is not going to make you a superhero, it's going to break you down.

As opposed to the popular belief that the modern professional world has ingrained into the psyches of most individuals today, relying on less sleep to get more work done is not a sustainable route to success. This has been proven so many times, and the lives and routines of some of the most successful individuals in the corporate world today vividly illustrate this fact. Perhaps one of the most important factors determining long-term productivity is constant and stable uninterrupted sleep.

Sleep is not all about the time period spent in bed, it's about the stretch of time spent sleeping without any interruptions. Having a minimum of 6 hours of undisturbed sleep constantly has been proven to improve memory, boost productivity and help improve an individual's health in the long term. Insomnia and constantly broken sleep have been known to lead to reduced productivity, poor memory and impaired mental abilities. To prove this fact, a scientific study was conducted in California, on a group of working-class adults. Half of the group were subjected to long, but interrupted sleep, while the other half were subjected to short, but undisturbed sleep. The latter group turned out to be more efficient and productive in handling their daily tasks than the former group.

Therefore, to get great sleep and boost your efficiency and productivity, it is not compulsory for you to go to bed at exactly 9 pm and wake up at 4 am. What is important is for you to:

- Have uninterrupted sleep as constantly as possible.
- Go to bed and wake up at the same time every day, and;
- Sleep for at least 6 hours on a daily basis.

Going to bed and waking up constantly at the same time on a daily basis helps to get your body in tune with your natural circadian rhythm. This helps your body to actually get accustomed to settling down at a particular time every day and improves the process of tissue repair and memory improvement. The key thing is for you to find sleeping and waking times that help you to maximize your use of your day. If you tend to get more done very early in the morning, you may consider sleeping early and waking early to get down to work immediately. If you tend to feel slightly disoriented in the morning, you may work till very late in the night and then wake up a bit late. It all depends on finding a pattern that works for you.

Still, it is important for you to get at least 6 hours of sleep regardless of what time you choose to sleep and wake and optimize your bedroom conditions to prevent interruptions to your sleep.

To prove that less sleep does not always equate massive success, the sleep statistics of some of the world's most successful individuals will now be reviewed.

Jeff Bezos is a household name in the E-commerce industry, and the CEO of Amazon has delved into manufacturing digital devices, creating a streaming channel, and establishing an online publishing platform over the years. The richest man in the world sleeps for 7 solid hours every day. He goes to bed at 10 pm and wakes up to make the most of his day by 5.

Bill Gates is the founder of Microsoft, the most revolutionary software company of the past century. Gates understands the importance of a good sleep pattern to productivity and long-term intelligence, so the software magnate goes to bed by 12 am and wakes by 7 am. He has probably figured that getting up in the wee hours of the morning does not always work for him, so he sleeps at midnight and gets up a little late to tackle his daily routine. Tim Cook, Apple's brilliant and revolutionary CEO, also sleeps for 7 hours a day, hitting the sack at 9:30 pm, and getting up by 4:30 am to attend to his responsibilities.

Amazon, Microsoft and Apple are three of the biggest companies in the world. Do you really think it's a coincidence that the men at the helms of affairs of these tech giants all get 7 hours of sleep consistently every night? I don't think so. Sleep is a really important factor contributing to success, and it must not be overlooked or compromised.

Barack Obama, America's first African-American President, Jack Dorsey, co-founder of Twitter and CEO of Square, Mark Zuckerberg, Facebook's young CEO, and Ellen DeGeneres, one of the most successful TV hosts of the 21ˢᵗ century so far, are all sterling examples of how a healthy and consistent sleep pattern can be a major contributing factor to long-term success and productivity. All these individuals get at least 6 hours of sleep every night consistently and try to go to bed and wake up at the same time every day. If maintaining a healthy sleep habit worked wonders for some of the world's most successful people, then why should you deprive yourself of sleep?

Some leading entrepreneurs do not just recognize the need for appropriate and sufficient sleep, they have experienced firsthand, how devastating sleep deprivation can be, and are now advocates of healthy sleep habits. Two of these entrepreneurs are Tesla boss, Elon Musk, and co-founder of the infamous Huffington Post, Arianna Huffington. Musk, who also runs SpaceX and SolarCity, has experimented with trying to achieve more by sleeping less, and he confesses that it didn't turn out great. Instead of achieving more, he ended up achieving way less than he could have. He observed that mental acuity tends to drop when certain sleep thresholds are unmet.

Arianna Huffington, on the other hand actually collapsed after trying to work for eighteen hours every day for a couple of days. After passing out from exhaustion and intense sleep deprivation, Huffington has learnt the importance of sleep to the body's proper function, and now sleeps at least 6 hours per day.

Some individuals, however, have been found to possess a special gene that allows them to perform efficiently on less sleep. Some people have also grown, out of habit, to be accustomed to sleeping for fewer hours and thus, perform efficiently even on as little as four hours of sleep per day. It must be noted that the fact that you know someone who performs brilliantly at work but sleeps for only four hours per night doesn't mean you should do the same. Sleeping for four hours might have been ingrained in the person's body physiology, or the person has a special gene called the 'Thatcher gene' that allows the person to sleep for less time than the average recommended period. Popular successful individuals who are known to sleep for less than five hours per night on an average include US President Donald Trump, who sleeps from 1 am to   4 am, and Chrysler Fiat CEO, Sergio Marchionne who wakes up every day at 3:30 am and has been reputed to have created the '8th day of the week' due to how much time he spends working. The important thing to note is, exceptions to the general rule guiding sleep and productivity may exist in your environment. That doesn't mean you should try to copy these people. They may have spent their whole lives surviving on little sleep, or they may just be genetically capable of performing excellently on little sleep. Individuals differ, so you do not have to compare yourself to others.

However, because these messages seem logical, and they are being passed all over the internet, people are beginning to see them as normal and true. People are beginning to feel ashamed; to feel like losers for sleeping 6 hours per day. They want to be like their favorite motivational speaker who screams into the camera on YouTube, telling them to only sleep three hours and grind like their lives depend on it.

The truth is, hard work is very important. Perhaps, the most controllable factor in the success of an individual is hard work. If you work hard, stay focused and dedicated to your goals, take out time to develop yourself, you are likely to achieve amazing results in your career, your academics, your business, and even your relationship, depending on exactly what you are dedicating your time and effort too. So, the motivational speakers telling you to work hard and put in the hours are not completely wrong, However, what the motivational speakers do not tell you, is that there is more to success and spectacular results than just sitting behind a desk, glaring into a computer screen for 21 out of 24 hours in a day. Success in life is about BALANCE. Once balance does not exist, everything begins to crash, and then everything eventually goes up in flames.

Because a lot of people are being misinformed that for them to succeed, they have to work harder and sleep less, more people are actually finding it extremely difficult to make headway in their careers. More people are frustrated with the slow progress of their businesses. Students are wondering why their grades still remain below average even though they are staying up all night almost every day of the week to make sure they consume as much materials on their courses as possible. The problem most of these people have in common is that they are not getting enough rest, hence, their bodies and minds are not performing up to their expected potentials.

Now, imagine a situation where a software engineer, for instance, instead of following all the misleading motivational messages found on most social media channels, actually works hard, not only just to achieve his career goals and complete assigned projects in record time, but also to ensure that his body gets enough rest to get it ready for every new day of work. Research shows that the daily productivity of such a professional could rise by up to 50% if the person actually switches to a healthy lifestyle that affords him the rest he actually desperately needs. So, while over-sleeping is bad, getting enough sleep is incredibly important, and is not an activity that should be overlooked.

You must have heard this for dozens of times, but according to medical research, for the human body to actually function optimally on a day-to-day basis, the average individual needs between 6 to 8 hours of sleep on a daily basis. That means you should go to bed somewhere between 10 pm and 11 pm, and wake up sometime between 5 am and 6 am to get ready for your day. If you actually can stick to this kind of rhythm, you would achieve more within the 16 – 18 hours you would be spending awake than you could ever achieve by staying awake for 20 hours. Think of the situation like this – the human body is like a car. A car needs fuel, oil, lubrication and a couple of other inputs to keep functioning optimally. Now, instead of buying premium-grade fuel for your car and keeping the engine properly serviced and lubricated, you just load it up with sulfur-laden petrol and refuse to service or oil the engine. The car might keep going for a while, but at a point, it will give up on you. It might be in the middle of that early morning Manhattan traffic on your way to work. Eventually, that breakdown will cost you more time and money than keeping that car in great shape could ever have.

As for the human body, if you refuse to sleep, you might not break down immediately, just like the car. However, every day that you do not get enough sleep, your productivity will decline steadily, until one day when you will break down from the accumulated stress. You might have to spend a few days in the hospital recovering, and your days off will cost you a lot. So, why not just maintain your body properly, save yourself the stress, and actually achieve more by sleeping better instead of punishing yourself unduly and actually achieving less?

The crazy thing about sleep deprivation is that it has even more damaging mental effects than physical. Being sleep deprived makes you less productive than you normally would, and that makes you begin to think that you actually need to sleep even less to clear up the backlog of responsibilities hanging on your neck. Remember that this backlog of work was caused by sleep deprivation leading to lower productivity in the first place. You begin to spiral down this vicious cycle, getting less and less sleep until you finally break under the pressure of all the intense, unnecessary stress you are putting yourself through.

Sleep deprivation is an increasingly endemic problem in today's corporate world. The aim of this book is to help the average individual to find better ways to get great quality sleep without breaking the bank. This book contains a variety of techniques, methods, devices and software applications that have been tested and trusted by certified professionals to help individuals sleep better, and actually ultimately become more productive and efficient in the long run. Sleep is way more important than you think; your body is not a machine. So, maintain it, and watch your life improve tremendously. How about we get cracking?

IMPORTANCE OF HEALTHY SLEEPING HABITS

The importance of sleep in the maintenance of good health and optimum productivity in the long-term cannot be over-estimated. It is likely, however, that over the years, you would have heard this statement several times, albeit in different forms and from different sources. Sleep, however, is more than just a necessary obligation that must be practiced to keep your body healthy. Sleep is a tool, which if utilized efficiently, can vastly improve your career, memory, finances, intelligence, relationships – every single aspect of your life. Healthy sleep habits help to repair the tissues and cells of your body and keep your brain alert and attentive at all times. What exactly, then are the reasons why you need to sleep properly and appropriately then?

- **SLEEP BOOSTS CONCENTRATION AND PRODUCTIVITY**

During sleep, the body goes into a 'low-activity' state characterized by reduced brainwave frequency and steady breathing. Not having to keep all your senses alert gives your body and nervous system the chance to be rejuvenated. This ensures that when you wake, all damaged tissues would have been repaired, and the brain and body would be energized to tackle the rigors of a new day. Temporarily hibernating helps your brain cells to rest, and get a chance to be revitalized. A well-rested brain then ensures that you can achieve maximum focus and concentration when you need it. However, when you do not rest, apart from the fact that you would be extremely tired and weary, your brain would find it hard to concentrate, because it has not had the chance to be rejuvenated. You would be stressed, your body would ache, and your focus levels would drop considerably.

Therefore, to ensure that you are always mentally, physically and psychologically ready to achieve your daily goals, healthy sleep is an indispensable daily activity (or inactivity!)

- **REDUCED RISK OF OBESITY**

Medical research has shown that sleeping for a minimum of six hours per night may significantly help to lower the risk of obesity. We live in an age where a lot of people consume so much junk containing saturated fats and unhealthy processed sugars. Sleeping is a great way for the body to detoxify itself of fatty foods that can accumulate over time to cause obesity. However, when individuals refuse to get enough sleep, and still practice unhealthy lifestyle habits during the day, adipose tissues begin to accumulate, and before long, obesity sets in. So, if you are looking to lose weight, you might want to pay attention to nutrition, exercise and of course, healthy sleep.

- **INCREASED PHYSICAL ENERGY**

Professional athletes, military personnel, and other individuals whose daily responsibilities involve intense physical exertion are people who truly understand the inestimable value of sleep. Sleep is incredibly important to the repair of worn-out tissues and to the relaxation of sore muscles. Therefore, after a long day of physical activity, you need sleep to help you recuperate. Sleep doesn't only help you stay active mentally, it improves your endurance and energy too.

- **REDUCED RISK OF CARDIOVASCULAR DISEASES**

When the human body is asleep, a variety of detoxification and rejuvenation processes are carried out. A lot of these processes help to get rid of harmful materials from the body. Saturated fats and cholesterol-filled foods are consumed in tons by the American population alone day in, day out. These foods tend to accumulate in the blood, and then end up clogging important arteries, which are blood vessels from which blood is pumped out from the heart. If sleep can be combined with exercise and proper eating habits, however, these fats may be gradually reduced within the body gradually until they are fully burned out. However, if you are eating junk, exercising lackadaisically and still not sleeping, then your risks of contracting a heart disease shoot through the roof.

- **REDUCED RISK OF DEPRESSION**

Depression has been severally linked to stress, insomnia, sleep deprivation and lack of rest. It's pretty simple actually. When you sleep, you give your brain the chance to organize and reconcile your thoughts, and the body repairs itself. Even though you may still have things to worry about, feeling energetic and mentally alert will make it easier for you to confront your problems head-on instead of getting depressed thinking about them. During sleep, the brain also releases hormones that help you to generally feel more pleasant and cheerful. So, if you feel yourself constantly having negative thoughts or feeling hopeless, you may need to improve your sleeping habits.

- **REDUCED RISK OF GASTROINTESTINAL INFLAMMATION**

Because the body automatically detoxifies itself during sleep, healthy sleep habits actually help to reduce the risk of disorders of the gastrointestinal tract. When you do not get sufficient sleep, your body cannot focus on repairing tissues and removing dangerous substances from your system. So, the unsafe stuff that you have consumed simply remain lodged within your gut, and with time, they begin to elicit inflammatory reactions from the organs of your digestive system, leading to abdominal pain, vomiting, diarrhea, and in some cases, the development of ulcers. So, before you choose work or movies over sleep next time, think about how important it is for those harmful substances that might harm your digestive system to be expunged during sleep.

- **IMPROVED IMMUNITY**

Sleep has been proven to help repair and rejuvenate worn-out cells and tissues of the human body. The human immune system comprises of millions of cells – the white blood cells, the macrophages and monocytes, the lymphocytes and other cells that work in harmony to ensure that you remain protected from environmental hazards that can put your health at serious risk. However, after fighting pathogens from the environment, immune cells might get destroyed. To help boost the efficacy of the immune system, sleep is required to ensure the repair of damaged cells and the synthesis of new ones. Therefore, sleep also helps to drastically boost the body's immune system by aiding repair of damaged cells and the synthesis of new ones.

FACTORS AFFECTING SLEEP QUALITY

ROOM TEMPERATURE

The temperature of a room is the first and perhaps the most important changeable factor that influences the quality of the sleep that an individual gets. Room temperatures affect the quality of sleep more than most people can imagine. When you sleep in a hot room, you tend to sweat, feel sticky and generally uncomfortable. Your resting heart rate also tends to spike, meaning that you are likely to feel groggy even after sleeping for up to 7 hours. Sleeping in a hot room also makes you predisposed to waking up at the slightest provocation. Therefore, to ensure that you get a great night's rest, how can you work on your room temperature?

Actually, a variety of options are available, but your best bet is a split air-conditioning unit. Even though these units may be quite expensive compared to other temperature-regulating options, they are still your best bet in the long-run to help you sleep better and feel more energized every day. The great advantage of an air-con is that you can set the temperature needed depending on what works for you. So, if you feel Sixteen Degrees Celsius is perfect, you can stick to that. If you'd prefer something a little colder, perhaps Ten or Eight, then you have the liberty to do that too. Air-conditioners enable you to experiment with different temperature ranges until you find the exact absolute temperature that works for you.

If you have a partner or roommate who prefers slightly warmer temperatures while sleeping, then such an individual can use layered sheets or a duvet instead to keep out the excess cold. This is why choosing colder temperatures beats warmer ones. In an uncomfortably hot room, there is little you can do to improve the situation, but when the room is appreciably cold, then you can make modifications to suit yourself.

The first major way the temperature of your surroundings affects your sleep is a factor the National Institute of Health refers to as sleep calmness. This is how relaxed and serene your sleep is. High temperatures do not in any way translate to calm sleep; the sweltering heat will make you grossly uncomfortable, you would probably wake up twice or thrice before dawn due to the heat, you might get sweaty and itchy, and all through the night, your resting heart rate is likely to be disturbingly high. So, sleeping in heat affects the tranquility of your sleep, thereby making you feel exhausted in the morning.

The ease of falling asleep is another major sleep factor that is hugely affected by prevailing environmental conditions, majorly temperature. When you settle in bed to fall asleep, but the atmosphere is just too hot, you tend to toss and turn, and you just do not fall asleep in time. Due to temperature spikes, some people do not even fall asleep at all, they just stay up all night, feeling uncomfortable, and then when they get out of bed at dawn to tackle their daily tasks, they feel extremely lethargic and unproductive.

Sleep satisfaction is another factor that the prevailing air temperature in your bedroom affects. The satisfaction which you derive from your sleep is evident in how energized and alert you feel when you wake up. If you wake up feeling like you just didn't sleep well enough, then you might have to alter your bedroom's temperature to help you feel more satisfied with the amount and quality of sleep that you get.

Finally, another sleep factor that is greatly influenced by prevailing bedroom temperature is sleep adequacy. Sleep adequacy and sleep satisfaction are extremely close, but they are not quite the same. While sleep satisfaction deals with how satisfied and contented you feel about the quality of your sleep, sleep adequacy has to do with whether you feel that the amount of sleep you got is enough. When sleep quality is low due to high temperatures, when you wake, up, you will feel like getting more sleep. That's because the sleep you got was inadequate. Sleep inadequacy may be caused by falling asleep late and waking up too many times in one night. Apart from temperature, an uncomfortable mattress and inappropriate light intensity may also lead to sleep inadequacy. So if you wake up and feel really lethargic and unmotivated to the extent that you just feel like grabbing one or two hours more of sleep, then you may need to critically look at the temperature of your room.

A split air-conditioning unit is not the only device that can be used to reduce your room's temperature and improve sleep quality. A standing fan, a ceiling fan, and specific devices that can be attached to your mattress may also be utilized. Some of these devices will be reviewed later in the subsequent section.

LIGHT INTENSITY

The light intensity in the room is another factor that decides how well you sleep. In most homes around the world today, most people have switched to fluorescent bulbs and white energy-saving bulbs that emit light rays that have a wavelength similar to that of actual daylight. Now, the way the body's circadian rhythm (or sleep-wakefulness pattern) works is that during the day, daylight stimulates the body to stay alert and face our tasks squarely, and darkness causes our alertness levels to wane so that we can get the rest that we deserve and then wake up at dawn to start another day. However, these daylight bulbs force the body to stay awake even when it is time to sleep due to the wavelength of the light they emit. The major problem that these bulbs cause is that they prevent you from falling asleep in time.

So, the best thing to do is to make your room as dark as possible, make it pitch-black if necessary. Specialized curtains are sold which help to keep out as much exterior light as possible. You may want to invest in these curtains to help you get better sleep. If you must sleep with some light on, however, then it makes sense to buy traditional tungsten bulbs that emit yellow light instead. The light rays emitted by these traditional tungsten filaments are different from the ones emitted by the sun and these white fluorescent bulbs, thereby aiding you in falling asleep faster and having a better sleeping experience. The best thing to do, however, to ensure that you get high-quality sleep, is to turn off the lights, use blackout curtains and relish sleeping in total darkness. This will help to reduce brain activity to the minimum and help you feel energized and ready to tackle your day head-on when you wake up.

Specialized night lights may also be a good way to help you get enough sleep if you prefer them. A red bulb is also a great option; red bulbs have wavelengths that have been proven to encourage sleep and rest. A lot of individuals have also attested to the fact that eye masks can help to keep out excess light and help them get better quality sleep. Computers, tablets and mobile phones can also be set to night modes after dark to ensure that the body prepares to go to sleep as soon as darkness sets in. This process and its importance would be discussed later in the section.

SOUND INTENSITY

Sound is another adjustable factor that goes a long way in determining how well or poorly an individual will sleep; whether through the night, or for one or two hours during the day. As predictable, it is healthier and widely recommended to sleep in a quiet and serene environment rather than a noisy one. Noisy rooms have been proven to cause restlessness during sleep – you are likely to shift and move uncomfortably when the room you are sleeping in is not tranquil.

While the playing of specific sounds might be extremely helpful in helping you to fall asleep in cases where complete quietness is not possible,—or is not helping—nothing rivals sleeping in a dark, quiet, and still room. Hearing numerous sounds such as road noise is likely to keep you up and prevent the process of falling into a deep sleep from taking place. Even if you do manage to fall asleep, the noises are likely to interrupt your sleep intermittently, and you may wake up feeling exhausted and bad-tempered. Sleeping in a noisy area may also have long-term effects on your mental health. So, how do you address the problem of hearing unwanted noises when you sleep?

Well, a reliable option is the use of double glass doors. If the sounds are coming from outside the room you are sleeping in, the use of double glass doors van help to keep the noises out. If the sounds are filtering through the windows, then you might need to consider changing the glass panes on your window to sound-proof ones to ensure that your room gets as quiet as possible when you need to sleep. If you can afford it, getting your whole room soundproofed goes a long way in ensuring that you get amazing, quality sleep. The use of sound-deadening panels on the roof of your room is also an extremely helpful option. It helps to keep out sounds from above, thereby helping to keep your room conducive to rest and rejuvenation.

Another proven way to keep the sound levels in your room appreciably low is to keep as little hard materials as possible in your room. Hard, sturdy surfaces tend to encourage the bouncing of sound waves within the room, making the room generally noisier and less serene. So instead of keeping a lot of metals and glass surfaces in your room, settle for more of clothing and wooden materials instead. Sound bounces off plastered walls, tiled floors and glass pretty rapidly, making your room uncomfortable for sleep. So, if it is possible to make adjustments to the contents and surfaces within your room to reduce the transmission of sound waves, please do so, as it will go a long way in making you sleep better in the long run. Other devices such as white noise machines and earmuffs that have been proven to help reduce noise intensity will be discussed in subsequent sections.

SAFETY AND SECURITY

Another extremely important, yet frequently overlooked factor that can completely make or ruin a person's sleep is the feeling of safety and security. When you feel reasonably safe in your environment, your resting heart rate is lowered, and brain activity decreases. This helps you to fall asleep faster, sleep more soundly, and transition seamlessly from one stage of the sleep cycle to another. If, however, you are extremely worried or overcome with the feeling of trepidation that anyone might come in to attack you, or something might crash into your room, then you are not likely to sleep well in the long term. So, as much as possible, work towards living in a relatively safe environment. Even though most populated cities have high crime rates, if possible, find an apartment in an area with fewer robberies and crime. It also helps to invest in an efficient security system; it doesn't have to be expensive. It might be a simple alarm with a security code. That way, you can go to sleep peacefully without having the constant fear that anybody can break in and attack you looming constantly over you. So, have an alarm system, keep your doors locked, and if possible, live in a low-crime environment. You might not think the feeling of security is critical to your sleep quality, but taking steps to improve your personal safety while you are asleep is bound to go a long way in improving your   sleep   quality.

COMFORT

Closely related to the feeling of safety is the feeling of comfort. Feeling comfortable while sleeping goes a long way into helping you to fall asleep and helping you to transition seamlessly from one phase of the sleep cycle to another. Many people do not realize it, but the mattresses, pillows and duvets they are using are negatively affecting the quality of their sleep, and are thus making them less productive than they could actually be. To ensure that you are as comfortable as possible, choose a sturdy mattress that does not bend under your weight. Also, try to invest in a supportive bed frame and a good pillow that provides your neck with needed support. Adjustable pillows made with memory foams are a great choice, but you need to make sure that they do not get you too heated up during the night.

Prevailing room temperatures also play a huge role in determining how comfortable you feel as you sleep. Investing in great bedroom furniture to help you get better sleep is a necessity, so as much as possible, get rid of that mattress that is slowly damaging your back, and that old or hard pillow that's making your neck feel disjointed every morning. Invest in great mattresses and pillows and watch your sleep quality skyrocket.

Moderately heavy duvets can also help to provide you with warmth and comfort, especially on the cold nights. While it is important to ensure that your duvet does not get you too heated up to the extent that you can't sleep properly, using an appropriate duvet can give a feeling of support and warmth that helps to boost the quality of your sleep tremendously. So, if you can afford it, it makes a lot of sense to get a heavy duvet to help you become more relaxed and comfortable while you sleep.

HUMIDITY

The final major environmental factor that may affect the quality of your sleep that would be discussed in this section is the prevailing air humidity, and the purity of the air. If you live in an apartment where the air is constantly polluted by dust, smoke or other air pollutants, then falling asleep, and transitioning seamlessly from one stage of sleep to another might be extremely difficult. So, if you can afford it, it can be very helpful to get an air humidifier to help maintain a constant humidity level in your bedroom and to help purify the air in your bedroom. Humidifiers are great sleep-improvement products, and if used properly, an air humidifier can help to rapidly and drastically improve the quality of your sleep.

In extremely dry environments, air humidifiers can help to spray mists of water into the room at specific intervals to ensure that while you sleep, the air does not get too uncomfortably dry and parched; a factor that could really decrease the quality of your sleep. Air humidifiers also help to filter the air with the aid of efficient air filters, helping to keep out not only dust particles in the air, but also acrid, uncomfortable smells and of course microorganisms. The general atmosphere of most of the biggest cities is populated with microorganisms, including the ones causing cold and flu. As you know, catching a cold can prevent you from even falling asleep at all. So, if you find out that you are getting bouts of cold extremely often, then it might be time for you to get an air humidifier to keep your air pure, and the microorganisms out.

Air humidifiers actually do a bit more than just keeping the pure and humid, the regulation of the air humidity also helps to keep your skin healthy and hydrated. Air humidifiers also help you to cut down on power costs. This is because when the air in your bedroom is sufficiently humid, then you do not have to put so much pressure on your air-conditioning system. When the air-con system uses less power, you save money. Finally, air humidifiers also help to keep the potted plants and wooden furniture in your bedroom pristine. By constantly spraying the room with mists of water, the air humidifier helps to keep wood and plants constantly hydrated, lengthening their shelf life and preventing quick degeneration due to dryness.

SLEEPING TO WIN

DEVICES AND HARDWARE TO HELP YOU SLEEP BETTER

A lot of people might think its geeky or nutty to actually buy devices and equipment that help you to sleep better. Well, sleep is extremely important, and if you are investing in buying great clothes to look professional when you go to work, then it makes a lot of sense for you to also invest in equipment to help you sleep better to ensure that when you show up to work looking sharp in your crisp clothes, you also feel sharp, alert and ready to crush your goals on the inside too.

As we grow into adults, one hard truth life teaches us is that nothing is ever handed to you on a platter of gold. Everything has a price; life is a bit straitlaced. If you do not pay the price for something immediately, you can believe me when I tell you that you will eventually pay for it later. So, change your orientation about the importance of sleep, and realize that it actually makes a lot of sense to invest in equipment to help you get enough sleep every day, thereby making you feel better and making you more productive. If you want to become a more effective individual, if you want to cross the line between mediocrity and excellence, then you need to make some sacrifices; to put in some efforts that other people aren't.

Because overall success in life depends on being successful and effective on a daily basis, and because daily success requires productivity that arises out of getting adequate rest, getting enough sleep regularly inevitably becomes a key ingredient of success. Not getting enough sleep is not only going to wear you out day in and out. It will eventually prevent you from achieving your desired goals.

In this section of this book, equipment that have been tested and examined critically, and have been certified to actually be immensely helpful in helping you get quality and refreshing sleep every day would be examined. Some of these pieces of equipment help you track the quality of your sleep, providing a diverse range of data on the quality of your sleep to help you determine what lifestyle changes you need to make to improve a particular sleep quality metric to ensure that you actually have better sleep experiences in the long run.

It is not enough for you to just wake up and think: "Wow! I had a good night's rest!" That might be enough for most people. But you are reading this book because you want to step out of the 'ordinary' into the 'Extraordinary' zone; you want to initiate a paradigm shift that is capable of turning your life around dramatically forever. So, this means that you are going to be extremely meticulous about even the slightest details. Like everything worthwhile, the journey to getting great quality sleep that makes you feel well-rested and rejuvenated to conquer your daily goals with a beast-like readiness is not going to be easy. Many people might think that the journey to sleeping better is just going to be a walk in the park, since it's sleep that is being improved, and sleeping is seemingly the easiest thing in the world. However, that mindset is dead-wrong. Improving your sleep is going to be more challenging than just plopping into bed at a particular time, and trying to get out of bed at a particular time.

Improving your sleep quality, in the long run, will entail you making a lot of major lifestyle changes out of the bedroom. You will have to cut down on unhealthy food. You will need to cut down drastically on alcohol and hard drugs, or preferably, abandon them completely. You will need to exercise efficiently to keep your body in shape and energized. All these activities complement each other and help you to achieve better sleep. But I can assure you, getting all these things done will not be easy, especially if they are self-destructive habits that you have been practicing all your life. Remember that thoughts become actions, actions become habits, habits become character, and character becomes a lifestyle. So, if you have been practicing destructive habits that have been hampering your efficiency and productivity both at work and on the home front for years, now is the time to begin major lifestyle changes. Trust me, getting yourself to be a productive superhuman will take more than just sleeping. It is going to be a fierce battle, but if you are desperate for a drastic, meaningful change, you will keep fighting till you win.

The great thing about some of the devices that will be discussed in this section is their ability to give objective, fact-based data on exactly how well a person actually sleeps on a daily basis. When you wake up, the only thing you can say is whether you feel rested or exhausted, and since we are looking for dramatic results here, that just won't cut it. So while most of the devices will be to help you alter certain prevailing environmental factors to help you sleep better, some devices will be used to help monitor your progress on your journey to become a less exhausted, and more balanced individual.

Just like machines, biological systems function based on the principles of input to output. The inputs you put in your body or dedicate to your body; food, drinks, exercise, sleep, all eventually determine how well your body performs in the long run. So, as you read through this material, you need to resolve to not only work on sleeping better, but on improving the quality of every input you provide your body with. This will ensure that you get the best possible results, and an overall healthy and outstanding body that will work perfectly with a sharp mind to achieve your goals.

Getting quality sleep is not all about spending more time in bed. As a matter of fact, oversleeping is bad for you. So, the aim of this section is not for you to use these devices to get so much sleep that you neglect the aspects of your life. As has been continuously reiterated, the aim to help you strike a healthy balance among all aspects of your life to help give you a body and state of mind that supports the realization of your dreams. Now, we move on to the first type of device recommended to help you get better sleep.

SLEEP AND ACTIVITY TRACKERS

Sleep and activity trackers are your most important companions on your journey to ensuring great sleep and a more productive life. Sleep and activity trackers come in a variety of forms – some are rings worn on a finger, while some may be in the form of watches strapped to your wrist. The common property shared by these devices is that they can generally be synchronized to your smartphone to give results on how well you slept, and how much physical activity your body experienced while you were wearing the device. Some amazing sleep and activity trackers available in the market for purchase right now include:

- Fitbit Versa 2, a smartwatch that measures sleep quality and intensity of physical activity extremely accurately. The Fitbit Versa 2 also possesses an in-built Alexa voice assistant that enables you to dictate messages, make searches, and even set alarms and reminders.

- Beautyrest, a non-wearable sleep tracker that uses a measuring pad positioned underneath your mattress to measure the quality of your sleep.

- Emfit QS, a non-wearable sleep tracker that a measuring strip placed beneath your mattress to analyze how well you have slept. The measuring strip uses a sensitive compression sensor to accurately calculate the quality of your sleep.

- Withings Sleep, a contactless mat placed under your mattress to evaluate your sleep metrics. Withings Sleep also has home integration features that help you to automatically control conditions that affect sleep, such as turning the thermostat on or off.

Finally, the Oura ring, which will be the example to be discussed in this section. The Oura ring is a practical device that is worn around the finger and helps to calculate sleep metrics which are sent to a smartphone app. The Oura ring is the most preferable sleep and fitness tracker out there for now, because of its convenience of use, its seamless integration with digital devices, and its helpful suggestions.

THE OURA RING: A CASE STUDY OF AN EFFICIENT SLEEP AND ACTIVITY TRACKER

At first, the name 'Oura ring' probably reminds you of some sort of mysterious, historic symbol that will magically turn your life around. While the extremely efficient and smartly designed Oura ring will not give you magic powers, it could most certainly help you become twice as productive as you used to be before beginning to use it, if utilized judiciously. If that is not magic, then I don't know what is.

The Oura ring is a small, discreet ring that can be worn on any finger and helps to track important details about your sleep. When you wake up, you can sync up the ring with your smartphone and view all the important details about your night's rest. The Oura ring is supposed to be worn day and night because it is not only capable of tracking the quality of your sleep, it also has the ability to track your activities throughout the day to give you important details about your productivity and how you can, in turn, work on improving both your sleep and productivity. Apart from being an extremely efficient sleep and activity tracker, the Oura ring also actually functions as an elegant fashion accessory – it's guaranteed to add a unique and elegant touch to your appearance. Simply wearing the Oura ring can also make it possible for you to start informative and educative conversations with other informed people who are trying to use this incredible device to improve the quality of their sleep. The ring is offered in an exciting range of colours, from black to silver and diamond.

The Oura ring has also been optimized to work seamlessly with phones on the IOS and Android platforms, so it doesn't matter what smartphone you are using, as long as your phone is powered by at least an IOS 11 or an Android 6 Operating system, the Oura ring will work seamlessly with your phone to transmit important sleep and activity-related data to it.

So, what exactly are the components of the data that the Oura ring transmits to a phone? Well, first and most importantly, the Oura ring tells you exactly how much sleep you got at night, in hours. A lot of people have this illusion that the amount of time they fell asleep is the difference between the time they got into bed and the time that they got out of it. However, it is no news that a lot of people find it difficult falling asleep after settling into bed. Some people may take up to an hour after getting into bed to fall asleep. Some people may also wake up severally in the middle of the night, and it may even take these individuals considerable time to slip back into sleep after getting back in bed. Since it is not possible for you to ascertain exactly when you fall asleep and how much time you spent sleeping, if you actually want to objectively measure the exact amount of time you spent sleeping, it makes a lot of sense for you to use an accurate device to measure that time period.

Apart from just reliably telling you exactly how much time you spent snoozing, the Oura ring also informs you about how much time you spent in each phase of sleep. Contrary to most people's beliefs, sleep is not just one long blackout. Sleep occurs in stages. When you fall asleep, you slip gently into a light state of sleep where it is possible for you to wake up at the slightest disturbance—a slight disturbance, in this case, maybe the slamming of a door or the crashing of thunder. However, as you sleep for longer, you actually transition sequentially into deeper stages of sleep, getting to the REM (Rapid Eye Movement) stage of sleep at a point. The REM phase of sleep, as the name suggests, is characterized by Rapid Eye Movement, and it is the stage where dreams occur. In the REM phase, individuals are also quite predisposed to jerking awake, and that usually has extremely devastating consequences. When a person is awakened during the relatively deep REM stage of sleep, the person is likely to experience intense fatigue and exhaustion all through the day, greatly affecting productivity and general performance.

Towards the end of the cycle, you get into the deepest stage of sleep, which is characterized by sound rest and extremely low brain activity. However, you do not remain in the deep stage of sleep all through the night until you wake up either. At a point, you actually transition back to the phase of light sleep and then the cycle begins all over again. The average individual may have up to 5 to 6 sleep cycles in one night. One single phase of sleep in the adult human lasts between 90 to 120 minutes. In babies, sleep cycles may last as short as 50 minutes per cycle. Therefore, as we grow older, we tend to spend more time on independent sleep cycles.

The Oura ring also efficiently tracks your heart rate all through the night, presenting that information on your smartphone in the form of a heart rate variability graph. Using standard indices, you can actually determine if your heart rate during sleep is normal or abnormal, and you can see how heart rate changes are affecting the quality of sleep. Even though a lot of people do not pay attention to the heart rate variability metric, it is actually a critical piece of information, because it not only tells you about how well you slept, it is also a representation of your general state of health. If you consistently find out that your heart rate is abnormally high when you check your sleep statistics in the morning, then you might need to seek medical help. Lifestyle changes have been known to help reduce resting heart rates, such as decreasing the consumption of alcohol and generally maintaining a healthy diet.

The Oura ring is also enabled to monitor your body temperature during the night. The temperature of the human body tends to vary based on a couple of factors – environmental temperature, immune system activity, and others. How hot or cold your body is, will go a long way in determining how well you sleep. Generally, lower body temperatures tend to promote better sleep. So, the Oura ring helps you to determine your average body temperature while you sleep, and helps you to figure out if you need to alter the environment in which you are sleeping to guarantee lower temperatures and a healthier, more refreshing sleep.

After observing how well you are currently sleeping, then you need to get to work and research what each detail means. What does your resting heart rate say about your current lifestyle? What is the normal, healthy resting heart rate of an individual your age? Are you within the healthy bracket? If you find out that a specific variable is perfectly okay, then you don't need to work on that, you just have to focus on what needs to be improved upon. After a week of use at most, you should have started figuring out how specific lifestyle habits affect specific metrics that influence the quality of your sleep. On the days that you exercise well, you should be able to note how it affects some of your sleep metrics. On the days that you don't exercise at all, you should be able to observe the repercussions too. Then, on the days you do not eat healthily; perhaps, you ate a lot of junk food containing a ton of saturated fats, or you drank way too much alcohol, you'll also notice the sleep metrics that these unhealthy lifestyle choices affect negatively. The point of the first week of use is for you to identify how great your current sleep quality is, and how you can commence your journey to improving the quality of your sleep.

As you begin to adjust your lifestyle to improve your sleep-influencing metrics, you will find out that you generally begin to feel better, energized and more productive. It's simple logic, but we as humans just do not like making the sacrifices that need to be made to make our lives easier. As I stated earlier, the journey to gaining better quality sleep and becoming more productive is going to be a torturous one. Giving up an addiction like alcohol or smoking, for instance, will be extremely important for you to get the kind of results that you truly desire in your sleep. However, giving up addictions can be difficult battles that would take years to be won. So, take solace in fighting your personal battles day-by-day. Every day that you manage to live a healthy lifestyle that leads you to get better sleep is a win. So, take that win, and appreciate it.

As you keep making efforts to improve your sleep metrics, you need to begin to focus on exactly what works and what doesn't. If you were told that consuming more of a particular food would help to lower your resting heart rate, and you eventually find out that consuming more of that food does not lead to any significant or appreciable changes in your Oura ring readings, you can discard that advice and actually focus your efforts on strategies that can actually help to improve your life. So, make a decision to focus on what actually works, and leave what doesn't work behind. When trying to improve their lifestyles to get better results in the workplace and in other aspects of their lives, some individuals tend to get too eager for results that they start trying out everything all at once, and then, in the end, they end up overwhelming themselves, ending up right where they started and barely making any progress.

You do not want to overburden yourself with too many commitments all at once. So take it step by step. Begin with making efforts to improve one metric by picking up one simple habit, or giving up one destructive lifestyle habit. When you have that fixed, and it becomes a core part of your life, then you would notice that your sleep becomes tremendously better. Then, that win spurs you on to take on another challenge to make the quality of your sleep even better. As you keep moving from challenge to challenge, the resolve to make your life better gets progressively stronger, and you keep finding the will you need to keep pushing on.

How exactly does the Oura ring work? It's extremely simple, actually. On the inside of the ring, there are extremely sensitive Infrared LED sensors that can monitor the pulse of the arteries in the finger you are wearing the Oura ring on. The Oura ring is able to use pre-programmed algorithms to derive important sleep-related variables from the pulse being tracked on the finger. A specialized and highly-developed temperature sensor is able to deduce the body's temperature all through the period the ring is kept on.

However, the wonders of the Oura ring do not end there. The ring also has a 3D accelerometer that helps you to track your activity during the day. With the frequency of your hand movements in conjunction with other measured factors, the Oura ring is able to deduce exactly how much work you are getting done. Getting this value is very important because it helps you to link how well you are sleeping to how productive you are during the day, while keeping other factors constant. The accelerometer also plays an extremely important role in helping to maintain an activity-rest balance. It doesn't matter how much great sleep you are getting, if you are constantly working your body past its natural limits, you will still continue to feel stressed and burned out. While a couple of factors like regular exercise and eating good food may help to boost your body's tolerance levels, it is extremely important to keep in mind that you should strike a healthy balance between working and resting.

The Oura ring, according to co-founder and President of the Oura corporation, Petteri Lahtela, was developed as a response to the discovery of the link between chronic stress and onset of disease. When the body is overworked and fed with food containing low amounts of the nutrients that the body actually needs, and is still not properly rested, then constant fatigue and poor health are bound to set in. The body finds it difficult to fight the factors that cause chronic diseases, and soon an individual is battling with a life-threatening ailment. It is therefore extremely important for us, as individuals to start thinking about the long-term consequences of our lifestyle choices.

The most important metric that the Oura ring gives to tell you how well you have rested is the readiness rating. The readiness rating is displayed vividly as a percentage on the top part of your phone's screen when using the Oura smartphone app. The readiness rating is basically a measure of how prepared your body is to tackle the rigors of another day based on how great your night's rest was. Generally, a readiness rating of 80% and above means you have gotten an amazing sleep, and you are ready to go conquer your daily goals. A readiness score in the 70s means you need to make a few adjustments to your lifestyle to improve the quality of your sleep. Anything less than 70 means you need to pay very close attention to your personal habits to ensure that you sleep better and become more energized in the long run. Extremely low readiness ratings on the Oura app may indicate serious sleeping disorders that may require medical attention.

Based on all metrics measured to give the readiness rating – resting heart rate, breakdown of sleep stages, total time spent asleep, and others, the app also gives quality advice and suggestions on what you could do to get better results. Perhaps, you need to go to sleep a bit earlier, or reduce the room's temperature to help you get better sleep. The app also suggests an optimal bedtime for you based on your schedule and sleep pattern to ensure that you get the rest that you require.

If you are an alcoholic, the direct implication of even a glass or two of alcohol in the latter part of the day is that early in the night, when you go to sleep, your resting heart rate spikes. This reduces the quality of your sleep, as it prevents your body from settling into a calming and relaxing rhythm. That's why people wake up feeling terrible after a night of drinking – the drinks have prevented them from sleeping well. So, if you constantly get high resting heart rates on the Oura app, then it is an indication that you need to tone down on the alcohol and other self-destructive habits.

Sleeping late means you'll get less REM sleep. This directly translates to a general feeling of lethargy and exhaustion all through the day. This feeling can be immensely debilitating and can end up affecting your productivity massively. The Oura app points out how your late bedtime is affecting your REM sleep and eventually, your general productivity. It then suggests an appropriate bedtime to improve your sleep and your effectiveness at work.

The Oura ring is constantly undergoing scrutiny and examinations to ensure that it delivers the best possible results and helps users as much as possible to develop healthier and more productive lifestyles. The Oura corporation, therefore, has developed a second generation of the Oura ring which is even more sensitive and provides more accurate information about the sleep of every user. Even though there's a 9 to 12 week wait time for the Oura ring, within weeks of appropriate use, you would start seeing mind-blowing results. The Oura ring gained critical acclaim when Prince Harry of England was spotted donning it in Australia.

Since the Oura ring helps to show the quality of sleep an individual gets on a daily basis, it only makes sense for an individual to actually take spirited steps to ensure that he keeps getting better sleep as objectively presented by the Oura ring. Therefore, while the Oura ring is a great objective yardstick for measuring sleep quality, other hardware or items actually also exist to actually help people sleep better and improve their Oura ring ratings. Of course, the gadgets explained below can be used without an Oura ring, but the ring and its application are a great way to track your progress as you set out to improve your sleep, and in turn, your life.

WEIGHTED BLANKETS AND DUVETS

These items have been mentioned in the previous section when we were looking at comfort as a factor in determining sleep quality. Weighted blankets help to relieve anxiety and sleep disorders, and they may help autistic patients who have difficulty sleeping to sleep better. Weighted blankets, because of the support and comfort they provide, give the body and brain a feeling of calmness and relaxation. Buyers must, however, be careful to buy only blankets made of skin-friendly materials.

When purchasing a blanket or duvet, be sure to choose a moderately heavy one. That means you shouldn't buy a blanket or duvet heavier than 40kg. Having weight on you while you sleep helps to soothe your parasympathetic nervous system, thereby helping to calm you down, and giving you better quality sleep.

SLEEP MEMORY FOAM

The most important item to help you guarantee a good night's sleep is a great mattress. Memory foam-containing mattresses provide incredible support and actually adjust to your body weight and height to provide you a great sleeping experience tailored just for you. Adjustable pillows made out of memory foam are also quite helpful in helping you to fall asleep faster, and of course, getting you better quality sleep. It is important not to stack up pillows too high to prevent neck pain. Specialized cooling pillows are available on sale that prevent excess heat with the aid of a cooling gel on each side. You can adjust these pillows by unzipping them and taking out some of the foam to help you get the best fit for your personal sleep preferences.

THE BIOMAT INFRARED MATTRESS PAD

This incredible device helps you to benefit from the delightful goodness of Infrared relaxation and healing therapy. This pad particularly comes highly recommended by some of the best physiotherapists and chiropractors in the US. The Infrared rays are radiated through specialized amethyst crystals, helping to relax muscles and joints, and helping you to wake up extremely energized and alert. Commercially sold as the Professional BioMat 7000MX, this incredible device can single-handedly improve the quality of your sleep drastically within a few days of use. All you have to do is plug the BioMat into a wall outlet near your bed, place the mat between your mattress and your sheets, and enjoy the goodness of its highly-developed Infrared therapy. The BioMat is affordable, efficient and safe, and if you engage in work that involves a lot of physical stress, then this device may just be the solution you have been looking for.

SOFT SILICONE EARPLUGS

These affordable little pieces are truly life-savers. If you live in a congested area and can't modify your apartment to make it soundproof or silent enough for you to get enough sleep, then you can turn to soft silicone earplugs for help. Originally designed for swimmers, silicone earplugs fit snugly in your ear and actually adjust to the shape of your ear as you slip them in. This makes it possible for them to provide maximum silence as you sleep because no space is left open for sound to enter your ears. The silicone earplugs are reputed for the comfort they provide, and you can get a pack of these little miracles for as little as $4 online.

WHITE NOISE MACHINE

This machine helps you to sleep better by creating a stable, soothing background noise that helps to phase out all other noises emanating from the surrounding environment. Some people actually prefer falling asleep to the sound of white noise than sleeping in complete silence. The white noise machine can be programmed to produce six different types of background noise themes: Ocean, Summer Night, Pure White noise, Rain, Brook and Thunder modes. The white noise machine can also help when you need to focus, or when you need to meditate. The white noise machine doesn't only help you to fall asleep, it also helps to keep you asleep by facilitating smooth transitions from one sleep mode to another.

MOBILE TASK LIGHT

This fascinating device can be set to automatically turn on at a particular time. It beams light of a particular wavelength on to your face, signaling to you that it is time to wake up. Experts have mentioned that waking up to the glare of daylight (or light with a similar wavelength) can help to further boost the body's circadian rhythm. Plus, waking to a beam of light instead of the sound of an alarm encourages you to actually get out of bed to begin tackling your daily activities.

RHINOMED MUTE NASAL DILATOR

This amazing product is for people who snore heavily and experience obstructions in their nasal passages during sleep. The nasal dilator works by quietly pushing away congestion in the nostrils and freeing up space for convenient inhalation and exhalation of air. By preventing vibrations on the soft palate, the nasal dilator helps to curb snoring and improve the quality of a user's sleep.

BREATHE SLEEP INDUCER

This simple, yet efficient device helps people to fall asleep by taking users through breathing exercises that help to calm the body. This sleep inducer is made in the form of a belt that is worn around the waist. Following the direction of the belt, users can embark on tailored breathing exercises designed to help them fall and stay asleep.

OTHER HABITS TO HELP YOU SLEEP BETTER

In the section, we would be looking at other extremely helpful gadgets that can be used, and habits that can be practiced to ensure that you get the sleep that you require to be productive and super-efficient every day. These gadgets and acts have been proven to be able to help you sleep better even if you are stuck in an environment that is not conducive enough to support quality rest.

So, first and foremost, we'll be looking at other habits that can be practiced in addition to the ones that have been mentioned in previous sections to ensure that you get as much premium sleep as possible.

DECLUTTER THE BEDROOM

This point is extremely underrated, yet undeniably important.
Sleeping in an extremely cluttered room filled with items such as
clothing, electronic devices or even food does not facilitate the
serenity that aids sleep. So, the next time you take some hours out
to rearrange your bedroom, try to remove as many unnecessary
items from your bedroom as possible. Clothing and accessories
should be stored securely in the wardrobe beyond your field of
view. If you are going to charge your phone and laptop in the room,
keep them as far away from the bed as possible, so that you won't
be tempted to keep pressing your phone or laptop deep into the
night, thereby preventing yourself from getting the relaxing sleep
that you require. The bedroom should be as free as possible and
project an air of serenity and tranquility, not one of chaos and
disorganization. Watching several objects littering your room will
force your brain to stay active, and chances are you'll be tempted to
creep out of bed to touch or use one of the things within your line of
sight. So, do yourself a favor, remove everything that is not
absolutely necessary from your bedroom so that you can sleep
better.

A part of decluttering is also keeping work files out of reach and out
of sight. You have given your best all through the day, now, it is
time for you to rest. Do not jeopardize the chance to rejuvenate and
refresh your body by keeping work stuff in your bedroom. As a
matter of fact, if possible, keep your laptop out of your bedroom. It
may sound like a strange idea at first, but you will treasure this
advice if you stick to it in the long run.

Laptops and phones are not the only screens that need to be kept
out of the bedroom, or at least as far away from you as possible.
Other screens such as Personal Digital Assistants and Televisions
should be kept out too. In modern society, it has become a sort of

status symbol for people to install televisions in all bedrooms, including the rooms used by kids. This is not a healthy habit. Both adults and kids need their sleep, and kids are even more prone to stay awake watching movies and playing video games instead of getting enough rest to tackle their daily activities the following day. So, for the sake of your long-term productivity and efficiency, keep the screens out of the room. Even if you manage to keep the screens off at bedtime, if you are having a little trouble sleeping, you are likely going to be tempted to turn on the TV, and from there, you might end up not sleeping till daybreak. So, keep the television in the living room, please.

Bills, letters, receipts, and things that would tend to trigger memories and worries that might keep you from sleeping also need to be kept out of your bedroom. Out of sight is out of mind after all. So, if you want your desired peace of mind, do not keep items that can trigger unwanted worries in the bedroom. You will only stay up late, thinking. This will then prevent you from finding a viable solution to your problems when you wake up because you will feel too foggy and exhausted to find any practical solutions to your problems. So, to prevent insomnia, declutter your room, and keep the screens out.

PUT YOUR PHONE ON AIRPLANE MODE

In the previous point, the importance of keeping your room as tidy and sparse as possible was emphasized, and the need to keep screens out of sight was stressed. However, this point stands independent because of the incredible level of addiction people have with their smartphones these days. It's terrible, it's sickening, and it's honestly preventing a lot of people from succeeding in their careers. Now, I am not saying I am a saint. There are times we all slip off the wagon, but the point is, you must work as hard as possible to make sure that you break your addiction to your smartphone.

Regulate the periods you use your smartphone. It's okay to chat with loved ones, but at specific times. Only check social media accounts, and non-work-related emails only when you are free, not when you are supposed to be pursuing your career goals or sleeping. Even work emails should be classified in order of priority. Set a time to check all work emails, probably after your first round of work towards midday, so that your mails do not prevent you from getting started with work as early as possible in the morning. Respond to important emails at once and forget about them. Draw up plans to act on emails that require you to carry out a particular duty. Delegate duties that can be assigned to others so that you can focus on important things, and most importantly, discard irrelevant mails. People spend a lot of time on their mobile phones, and the sad thing is they spend the bulk of that time doing irrelevant stuff.

So to ensure that your smartphone does not get in the way of your sleep, it is advisable to keep it on airplane mode and charge it from a wall socket that is as far away from your bed as possible. That way, when it is time for your alarm to wake you up, you would actually have to get out of bed and walk to where your phone is to put off the alarm instead of just rolling over, hitting the snooze button, and going right back to sleep.

Still, on the smart use of your smartphone to prevent sleep deprivation, try to utilize the night light mode on your phone and laptop after dark hours. Depending on what time the sun sets in your location, you can set your night light to become automatically activated from around 7 pm to 8 pm. The light rays emitted by your phone in its normal mode tends to prevent you from sleeping in time because it has a wavelength similar to daylight. That wavelength passes a message to your brain that it needs to stay active because it is not time to sleep yet. So, if you need to use your smartphone after dark, switch on the night light to enable you to fall asleep faster.

CHOOSE DIM LIGHTS OR PITCH DARKNESS

In the last point, the usage of night modes on your smartphone and laptop was discussed. Earlier in this book, the importance of choosing tungsten bulbs over fluorescent and white energy-saving bulbs was also discussed. To further ensure that you fall asleep more easily, medical experts also recommend using a candle or a fireplace if you cannot bear to sleep in a pitch-black room. Candles and fireplaces light up your room with a warm, incandescent glow that soothes, relaxes and actually induces rest. So if you have a fireplace in the room, stack up that alcove with logs or coal and fire it up at night before bed. You will absolutely love the ambience the fire's glow will give the room, and of course, you will fall asleep more easily.

The reason why night lights on digital screens and fireplaces and candles are so super-effective in inducing relaxing sleep is the fact that they induce the secretion of melatonin, a hormone that is secreted by the pineal gland in the brain that helps to calm the body and encourage the body to go to sleep. The effect of yellow incandescent bulbs, night lights and candles and fireplaces on the brain is that they help the brain to feel calm and relaxed, thereby encouraging the secretion of this 'sleep hormone.'

White lights and daylight, on the other hand, encourage the secretion of cortisol, which is a hormone that facilitates activity and prevents sleep. So, there is actually a biological basis to the way your body reacts to lights of different wavelengths.

CLEAR UP ALL PRESSING ISSUES BEFORE BED

One of the most potent ways to give yourself insomnia is to go to bed without clearing out an extremely urgent problem that requires immediate attention. If it absolutely needs to be done before bed, then clear it up as fast as possible before hitting the sheets. It is recommended to get into bed early so that you can get enough sleep before daybreak, but it is obvious that getting into bed early won't do you much good if you are going to spend all the time you're supposed to spend sleeping thinking about an urgent task or a burning issue. So, make all urgent decisions and clear out all important exigencies that MUST be done during the day before going to sleep. That way, you will be able to go to sleep when you are done and actually benefit from the few hours of sleep you will get instead of rolling around in bed all night wishing you had attended to a file before leaving the office.

While following this rule, it is also important for you to remember that only extremely important issues that cannot be delegated or attended to the following day must be handled before bed. Once it's your bedtime, if that task or job can wait, then let it wait. As a matter of fact, it is advisable not to begin any fresh tasks after 7 pm. Finish up all you have to do, use the night mode if you have to work on a screen in the night, and settle in to sleep by reading a book or listening to calming music.

ESTABLISH A 2-HOUR WINDOW BETWEEN WORK AND SLEEP

Experts have advised that it does the body a lot of good to wind down naturally between work and bedtime. This winding down process allows the body to relax and ease off stress even before sleeping at all. Therefore, even if you cannot let go of two hours between finishing up work and sleeping, try to at least free up one hour between the close of work and your bedtime. This time window can be used for a variety of amazing tasks that most people claim not to be able to find time for bonding with a spouse and family members, or reading a self-development book. Whatever you choose to do within this 1 or 2 hours time frame depends on you, but make sure it is an activity that does not require extreme brainpower.

Also, within this time frame, just before bed, it is advisable to take a shower. Taking a shower before bed will not only help you to maintain relatively high personal hygiene standards, it will also help your body to feel relaxed and less sticky when you get into bed, thereby allowing you to fall asleep faster. Even if your room is a little hot, taking a shower helps you to remain a bit cool, enabling you to sleep peacefully through the night. So, don't just arrive from work, eat junk food, strip off your clothes and crash into bed. Put a semblance of order in your life and allow your body some time to gradually unwind before bed.

SLEEP FOR A MINIMUM OF SIX HOURS

As mentioned at the beginning of this book, motivational speakers are capitalizing on the demanding nature of the corporate world to force professionals and entrepreneurs into doing more work on a daily basis and getting less sleep in the process. Once again, it does not make you a loser to sleep for six to eight hours a night. As a matter of fact, it makes you a balanced individual who has a higher chance of actually building a stellar career because you will be more alert, productive and efficient at work. So ditch all the deceitful motivational speeches that tell you to sleep for three hours. Of course, it is important to wake up early so you can begin tackling your daily tasks head-on, but do not forget that waking early means sleeping early. Even if you have a very demanding job, try to carve out at least six hours (say, between 11 pm and 5 am) to get a refreshing night's sleep. By 5 am, you can hit the ground running because you will actually be rejuvenated to start going again. As you crush your workouts and prepare for work, you will feel the difference in your mental alertness and your physical readiness for work. If you sleep only three hours, trust me, you'll feel miserable all through the day and end up achieving less and less as you keep up that self-destructive habit.

Getting enough sleep also helps to improve your memory. During sleep, the body does not completely shut down, even though it remains in a low-activity mode, much like your laptop's 'Sleep' mode. However, during sleep, the body is still working, and it is during sleep that tissue repair and reconciliation of important thoughts and memories occur. This is why people who have important tests, exams and presentations are advised to get as much sleep as possible before the big day. So, don't compromise your sleep for work.

MAINTAIN CONSTANT SLEEPING AND WAKING TIMES

As we grow up and sleep and wake every day at fairly constant times, the body establishes a pattern known as the circadian rhythm. The circadian rhythm is what causes you to start feeling sleepy at a particular time, and what causes you to wake up around the same time almost every day. The circadian rhythm said to work in line with the setting and rising of the sun, but with habit, it may be adjustable. So, if you desire to get six hours of sleep every day, then endeavor to go to bed at a particular time, and you can begin by setting alarms for the time you decide to wake up.

A medically-proven fact is that it takes 21 days to adopt a habit and 90 days to turn that habit into a lifestyle. So, if you want your lifestyle to be sleeping by 11 and waking up by 5, then as much as possible, once it 10:45, slip into bed so that by 11, you can be asleep. This principle will not work if you slip into bed and start watching a movie or fiddling with your phone. Get in bed and sleep, and wake up to the sound of your alarm. As time goes on, you will find out that even before your alarm rings, you might already be awake and ready to tackle your day with full vigor. Following your body's natural circadian rhythm helps you to get better quality sleep and of course, be more effective and productive at work.

However, do not forget that if you can comfortably afford it, it is a lot more preferable to get a full eight hours of sleep every day.

DO NOT EAT AFTER 7 PM

I understand that you love your midnight snacks and drinks. I also understand that you've been indulging in midnight eating all your life. Well, guess what? It's time for a paradigm shift; it's time for everything to change. Eating late into the night has a lot of destructive effects, and while you might not be aware of the effects now, when you eventually quit late-night eating and start finishing up your dinner at least three hours before bed, you will actually begin to notice the differences. Eating late into the night grossly affects the quality of your sleep and how easily you drift into sleep.

Normally, during sleep, the body gets to work. The fact that the body is currently at rest gives it the opportunity to work on repairing worn-out tissues and reconciling thoughts to improve a person's memory. However, when you eat dinner by 12 am and crash 30 minutes after, your body will be forced to digest the food you just ate in your sleep instead of repairing tissues. Eating late will not only make it harder for you to fall asleep, but it will also make it difficult for you to stay asleep. Your body will be trying to digest the food you just consumed, which means it will not be able to fully rest and carry out tissue repair. That means you are likely to snap awake multiple times during the night. During the light phases of sleep, you may even feel stomach upsets. Eating late may seem like fun, especially when you are having friends over, but it does no good for your health. Keep the late-night snacking to a bare minimum and watch yourself gradually begin to feel more energized and alert in the mornings. Due to the fact that your brain will also be able to settle down and reconcile all thoughts and memories processed during the day, you will find out that you actually tend to remember important pieces of information faster when you allow your body to truly rest when you go to sleep.

So eat your dinner by 7 pm, or latest by 8. Allow the food three hours to digest, and then go to bed. As much as possible too, do not eat heavy foods for dinner that will take too long to be digested. Choose easily digestible foods like veggies, salads and fruits. Eradicate saturated fats and heavy carbs from your dinner schedule; they are bad for you.

Closely related to not eating late is reducing your alcohol intake, especially towards your bedtime. The ideal thing to do is to start working on quitting alcohol, tobacco and any hard drugs altogether if you are using any, because these substances tend to damage more than just your quality of sleep over time. Excess consumption of alcohol has been linked to serious liver problems and even heart disease. When you consume even just a glass of alcohol before bed and you check the Oura app on your smartphone in the morning, you will find out that your resting heart rate would be high, at least in the earlier parts of the night, compared to the times when you didn't drink at all. So, cut down on the alcohol and all other harmful substances. Your future self will thank you for your sacrifices.

These are all the habits that will be covered in this section. Remember that this is by no means a completely exhaustive list. You can carry out your own personal research to find out other helpful practices that can help improve the quality of your sleep in the long term. As you implement these practices, be sure to check out their effects on your sleep by looking up the statistics displayed by your Oura ring every morning. Remember that the ring helps gives an objective breakdown of the details of your sleep. So, while you may feel excited that some herbal root extract you had gulped the night before had helped you to feel stronger in the morning, check your Oura stats first. If the extract improved your readiness rating by reducing your resting heart rate or your body temperature, then you can inculcate it in your diet. If it raised your blood pressure or resting heart rate, don't use it again.

SCENTS AND FRAGRANCES

Since time immemorial, aromatherapy has been used for a lot of stress-relieving and healing processes, including inducing sleep. You can also benefit from the massive benefits of aromatherapy to get better quality sleep and feel more energized and alert every morning. Essential oils, fragrances and pure extracts may be sprayed into your room or onto your pillow to help you get the sleep that you need. Fragrances have been proven to have a wide range of health benefits including:

- Easing restlessness and agitation (Lavender)
- Decreasing heart rate and lowering blood pressure (Vanilla)

- Enhancing moods and performing antidepressant functions (Vanilla and Lavender)
- Increasing the brain's delta and theta activity, thereby promoting sleep (Valerian)
- Easing sleep disturbances and allergies (Sandalwood)
- Relieving fatigue, nervous exhaustion and menstrual pain (Juniper)
- Lowering cortisol levels and managing psychological stress responses (Bergamot)
- Killing bacteria, viruses and fungi (Ravensera)
- Improving overall daytime functioning and productivity (Chamomile)
- Cleansing the immune and lymphatic system (Geranium)
- Easing physical pain and tension (Rose)

Note that some of these scents may be used in specific combinations to have even more powerful effects.

SOFTWARE APPLICATIONS TO HELP YOU SLEEP BETTER

In this section, to wrap up this piece, we would be looking at helpful software applications and programs that can be used on smartphones and in some cases, personal computers that can be utilized by individuals who desire better long-term sleep quality.

OURA APP

This application works in tandem with the Oura ring described extensively in the first section of this book to help users to measure the quality of their sleep objectively using a couple of standard metrics. The Oura application works smoothly on Android and IOS platforms and has a brilliantly designed user-friendly interface. The application interpolates sleep and activity-related data from the night before and the day before to give a measure of how biologically prepared an individual is to tackle the challenges of a new day. This overall rating is displayed vividly at the upper part of your smartphone's screen and is called the readiness rating for the day. As mentioned earlier in this book, a readiness rating of 80 and above means you have gotten an amazing night's rest, and are ready to fully tackle your day head-on. A reading in the 70s means you have to sleep earlier or make a couple of minor changes to your work and sleep habits to help you sleep better. A readiness rating in the 60s and lower means you have to make major changes to effect the change that you desire in your sleep quality and overall productivity.

As has been reiterated severally, there is no point in using the Oura ring and the smartphone application if you have no intention of actually committing to making the tough lifestyle changes that will help improve your sleep quality and the overall quality of your lifestyle. The whole point of the application is for it to display your current sleep statistics and advise you on how to improve those individual statistics. If you buy the ring and install the application and still do not make concerted efforts at improving your statistics on a daily basis, then you might as well not have bought the ring at all. If you are trying to improve your REM ratings for instance, then you should be considering making your environment more conducive to sleeping by sound-proofing and turning out the lights. You should also try sleeping earlier.

If you are trying to improve your resting heart rate on the other hand, then cutting down on stress, alcohol, unhealthy foods may just be your way out. Working on perfecting one metric at a time will help you to take giant strides on your way to become an incredibly effective individual.

The Oura smartphone application also comes with a cloud storage platform that helps to store all your daily ratings, examine trends of how well you have improved or regressed since you have been using the Oura ring, and predict how better you can get if you keep up your current efforts geared towards improving the quality of your sleep. To access the cloud storage platform, you are required to log on to cloud.ouraring.com. You would need your e-mail address and a password to log in. Once that's done, you can access your stored data, monitor your progress from your online dashboard and make plans to improve on your flaws, and of course, boost your strengths. There is also the default view that provides your newest sleep data.

The main Oura ring app has an all-day guide that tracks your activity data during the day and allows you to share your readiness and activity data with selected friends. That way you and your committed friends can work together towards achieving your common goals of better sleep quality and productivity. The interface of the Oura ring application is divided into the Main View Timeline, the Bedtime Window, the Notes and Tags section and the Trends View.

The main view timeline is the first and most important section of the app interface. It's easy to read, with an elegant and vibrant, yet minimalistic style. The main view timeline helps you to track activities that affect your sleep and productivity such as the time you get to sleep and the time you wake up. Your readiness score is displayed as a bold figure on top of the main view timeline.

Right below your readiness score on the main view timeline is a summary of the important data pertaining to your previous night's sleep. In this section, you will be able to access information about exactly how long you slept, and what exact times you slept and woke. Tracking this information over an extended period would let you have a clear picture of your body's normal circadian rhythm. In the summary section, you will also access information about how much time you spent on each stage of sleep.

The next element on the main view timeline is the Activity target element. This element helps to match the quality of your rest to how productive you are at work, and helps to tell you if you need to push yourself harder, or if you require a break. For extended information about your activity data, you can tap the activity card and explore the available options. Going through your activity data will enable you to realize how much work your level of rest allows you to actually achieve.

After the Activity target element comes the Tags, notes and Manual Activity inputs. Here, you can use tags as single words to remind yourself of what you need to do, information that needs to be researched, or things that you need to stop. Notes are a bit more comprehensive than tags, and they allow you to actually record your plans within the app so that you do not forget them. In the manual activity inputs, you have the liberty to record what you were able to achieve in a day, and correlate your level of productivity to your sleep quality over a period of time.

The last section allows you to track restful moments within the day, perhaps the time when you opted for a power nap. Restful moments are tracked by monitoring your resting heart rate.

BEDTIME WINDOW

The bedtime window is the second component of the Oura smartphone application interface. This section gives you information about your circadian rhythm, reminding you when it's time to sleep, and when it's time to wake up. The Oura app follows your activities and sleep and wake times to gauge your lifestyle and give you the best suggestions to optimize your productivity.

Insight cards are available to provide you with details of your readiness data – your resting heart rate, your heart rate variability and body temperature deviations during the night. The expanded insight section also gives a night heart rate variability curve to let you note exactly how your resting heart rate spiked and dipped during the night. A graph is also plotted to illustrate your average nocturnal respiratory rate. This tells you how heavy or shallow your breathing was all through the night, and if you need to make some adjustments to your sleeping conditions or see a doctor.

In the sleep card section of the bedtime window, you are able to access information about the quality of your sleep, time spent asleep, sleep efficiency percentage, average resting heart rate, sleep stages and cycles completed and the time you spent awake.

Below the sleep card is your activity card. In this section, you get to access details of your personal activity data such as activity goals, calories consumed and burned, distance walked in steps and in kilometers, time spent in sedentary mode, and the intensity of your activities and their effects on your vital signs. You can, of course, share all this information with your partners in progress and see how their activities are promoting their overall productivity and health too.

TRENDS VIEW

In this section, you can access daily, weekly, and monthly readiness trends, and monitor how your lifestyle is affecting your sleep and productivity. Using the trends view, you can follow how the efforts you are putting into changing your lifestyle are paying off, what areas you still need to work on, and the areas in which you are deteriorating.

Overall, the Oura smartphone app is a wonderful companion to the Oura ring and is one of the singular most helpful sleep-improvement software applications available in the market right now. It's extremely user-friendly, offers helpful advice and shows you, objectively, exactly how things are so you can get to work on improving your sleep, and eventually, your life.

CUSTOMIZED HEALTH TRACKING SHEET

A lot of people might think spreadsheets are only helpful for financial analysts and mathematicians. Well, that's wrong. Just like Word processors, spreadsheets are for everyone; they serve as an efficient means of presenting stored information recorded over a period of time, and of course, help to make critical decisions from the recorded information. Using the Google or Microsoft Excel spreadsheet program, you can design your own personal health tracking spreadsheet and use it for a year-round tracking of your sleep statistics and improvements. How do you design your own personalized and efficient spreadsheet? It's pretty simple.

On the first vertical column on your left, list the months of the year, starting from the second row of the first column. Leave the first box bare. Starting from the second box on the first row, list the different metrics measured by your Oura ring, and then add a couple of other metrics that would be judged based on your own daily personal opinions. These metrics would be subjective, of course, but they would be used to compare your actual feelings to the readings from the Oura ring.

The Oura ring statistics that would be included in the top row of your spreadsheet would include the time you go to bed every day, your wake-up time, total sleep duration, time spent awake, time spent in light sleep, time spent in REM phase, time spent in deep sleep, average heart rate, low resting heart rate (LRHR), low resting heart rate time (LRHR time), body temperature, respiratory rate and heart rate variability. You can simply copy these statistics right from your Oura software app to your spreadsheet.

A separate metric known as timing is recorded after heart rate variability. This metric helps to measure how strictly you stick to your natural circadian rhythm. If you sleep at the same time and get up at the same time every day, you get a perfect average monthly score of 100% for timing. If you deviate widely from your normal circadian rhythm, then you get a low timing percentage. If your sleeping and waking times vary too widely, your productivity is likely to be affected, so the importance of this metric is to help you have a fairly regular pattern for sleeping and waking.

The last Oura ring column will be for your daily readiness scores. With the aid of the spreadsheet, you can determine your weekly and monthly averages for readiness, and focus on building habits that help to improve your daily readiness and productivity.

After readiness comes the metrics that will be judged by your personal opinion. The first metric in this section is Alertness, and this is dictated by how prepared and ready to tackle the day you feel when you wake up. Alertness in the morning is usually greatly affected by sleep satisfaction, sleep adequacy and time spent asleep. You can rate your alertness as a percentage and type it into the appropriate box for the day. The next metric is the mood metric. How great do you feel when you wake up? Do you feel motivated and super-eager to burst out of the house and start crushing your goals for the day? Do you feel like just going to work and getting things done so you can come back home? Do you feel like not even going to work at all? These feelings are dictated by your mood, and you can use how you feel every morning after sleeping to rate your mood.

The next metric is the soreness metric. How sore do your muscles feel when you wake up. Does your body feel weak and tired even after a long night's rest? If you are the kind of person that works out, do your muscles feel strained? Your soreness level can be recorded in the appropriate box for the day. The next metric is 'Meditation time.' In here, you record how much time you spend meditating in the morning. The recommended time for this is 20 minutes. Meditation has been proven to help clear the mind, improve motivation and make you feel generally more favorably disposed towards crushing your daily goals.

The next metric after meditation time is the diet metric. How well are you eating? Are you eating loads of junk and unhealthy carbs and fats? Are you sticking to a good meal plan of proteins, vegetables and fruits, with less fats and carbs? Rate how well your dieting in the past 24 hours has gone in this box. It will constantly remind you to strive to stay true to your dieting and body goals. Dieting has been proven to not only be great for a person's health and mental clarity, but it has also been proven to improve mental strength and personal discipline. You are literally keeping yourself from eating sweet and attractive things that you can afford, but can be deleterious to your health. It takes a high level of mental strength to do that, and the longer you stick to your dieting plan, the stronger your resolve becomes. If you completely stuck to your dieting plan, you can rate yourself a 1. If you managed but snuck in a snack or two, give yourself a two. If you completely went off the rails and ate what you weren't supposed to, then you get a three. That means you have to improve your resolve and determination to eat healthily.

If you are the type of person that takes supplements, you can name your next metric 'Supplements.' If you take your meal supplements, you get a 1. If you don't, you get a 2. The next metric is the Workout metric. In this section, using a 1 for YES and a 2 for NO, you record whether you exercised in the past 24 hours. The next three metrics are inter-connected. The first one is the time you start work, the time you finish work, and the total period spent at work. Of course, this metric is meant to be filled in at the end of the day after you must have finished working.

The next metric measures your personal work output. How much were you able to achieve compared to your actual plans? Your output rating is meant to be measured as a percentage. The next metric is also to be measured as a percentage, and this is your Focus rating. How focused were you at work? Rate yourself over 100.

The next metric encourages you to plan for tomorrow from today. If you planned ahead for the next day, then in this metric named (PLAN TT) you write a 1. If you didn't, well, you give yourself a 2 and remember to carry out this responsibility the next day. You can also add a metric column for reading. Did you read during the day? If you did, type in 1. If otherwise, you get a 2. For all YES/NO questions, you can also fill in 'YES' or 'NO' into your spreadsheet if that would make things clearer and easier to work with.

Finally, the last metric should be named Audit. This metric is not to be filled by you; it is to be filled by someone you are accountable to. This person checks your overall performance and keeps you in check to make sure that you fill in your spreadsheet every day so that you can monitor your performance by yourself. Auditing may not be possible on a daily basis, but ensure that it is done at least once per week. When you know that someone is going to be checking up on your records, you will be more motivated to fill them. If there are any notes for a particular day that need to go into the record, then you can put them under a 'Notes' section. If you were sick for instance, you can note it here as a reason for possibly poor metrics.

At the end of the week and the month, you can calculate your performance average and figure out aspects of your life that you need to work on, both based on your personal opinions and the objective data of the Oura ring.

The aim of the spreadsheet is to make sure that you never fall off the wagon while working towards living a more relaxed and productive life. Within a month of using the amazing method that has worked brilliantly for lots of entrepreneurs, professionals, students, sportsmen and politicians, you would be glad you made the big first effort of starting it.

FINAL NOTES

There is no point in gaining information that you do not put into practice. The aim of this book is not to just provide you with information about products, techniques and habits that can help you sleep better, the aim is to help you initiate a drastic turnaround in every aspect of your life – your finances, your academics, your relationship, your health. So, this book may be a guide, but ultimately, the power to make the powerful secrets in this book work for you rests solely in your hands. Decide for once, to actually act and take a step to make your life a better one. If you manage to inculcate the habits present in this book, you will definitely become productive enough to be able to create time to learn more, and finally move your life from where it currently is, to where you are meant to be.

Once again, I am using this medium to welcome you to a more efficient and productive world filled with infinite possibilities. As you begin to implement the techniques in this book, I say to you: "Godspeed!"

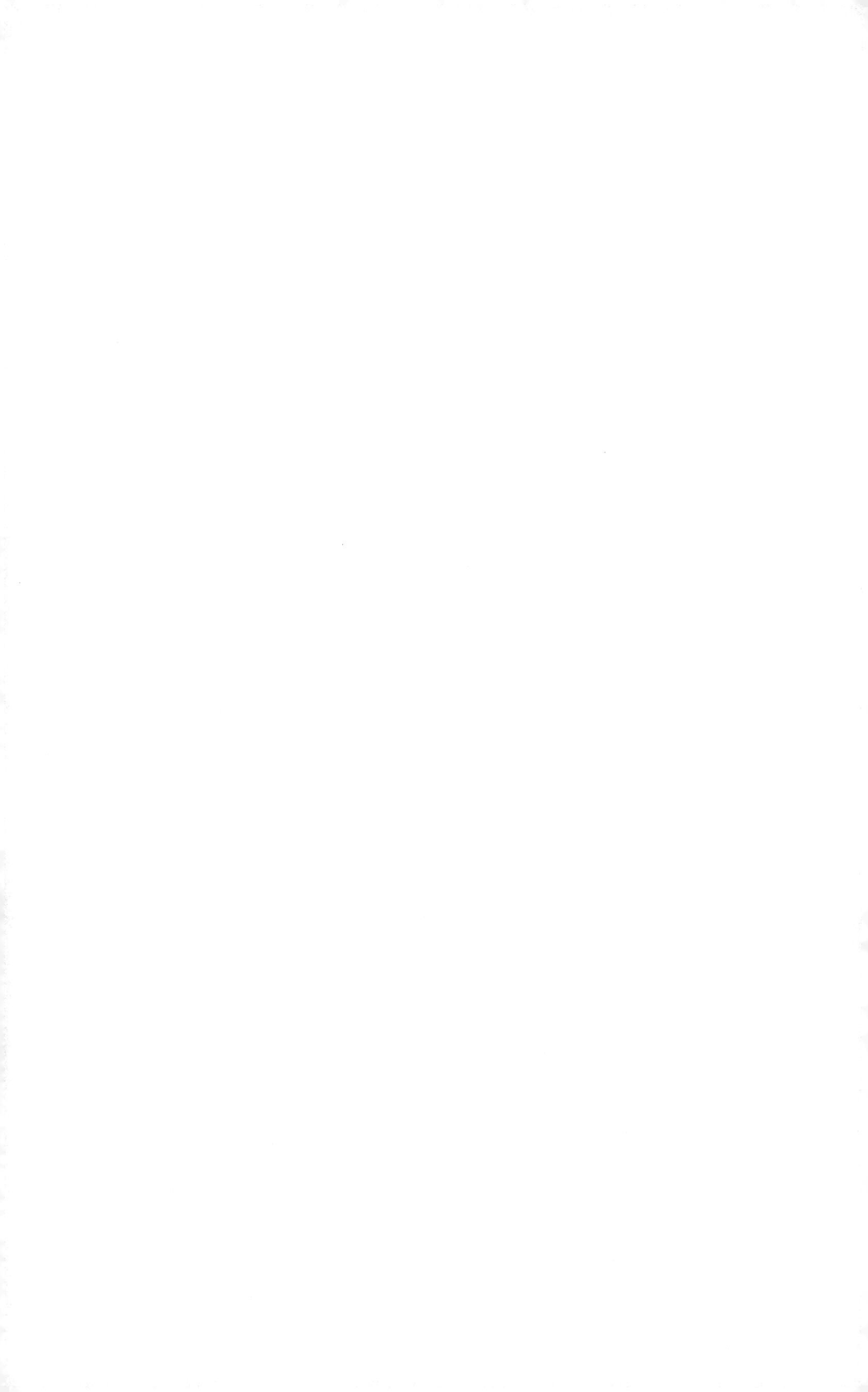